Illness Addiction

A companion guide for health promotion in substance use disorder

Authors:

Dr Gargi Sinha

MBBS (LHMC, New Delhi, India), PGDACP (India)

Master of Public health (Edith Cowan University, Australia)

Public Health Researcher in Addictive Behaviour

Dr Nilotpal Das

MBBS, MD Psychiatry (AIIMS), DNB, MNAMS, FRANZCP

Foreword

While the medical model of addiction addresses the harmful effect of drug and alcohol on a single patient only, however, public health strategies have aimed to discuss prevention, reduction and support for an individual, family and community, using various approaches such as harm minimisation approach. The overarching term of harm minimisation encompasses three different pillars to address the problem of excessive use of drug and alcohol in a community. These three pillars are demand reduction, supply reduction and harm reduction.

Broadly, the range of preventive and supportive community programs falls in the bracket of demand reduction. Interestingly, investing in preventing early uptake and treatment programs can address the problem of drug and alcohol in a community in an evidence-based approach. However, policymakers focus solely on supply reduction that aims to stop drug and alcohol by taxation and law enforcement agencies such as police and border control. As a result, people suffering from the problem of addiction often trapped in the cycle of breaking the law and stigmatised completely by society and lawmakers. Unfortunately, there is a vast gap that exists in low resource setting of India to adopt harm reduction approach that aims to minimise the harmful consequences of drug and alcohol use to an individual, family and community.

To understand the dilemma of a person and a family suffering from addiction, one needs to understand the nature of the addictive substance. There are several books available for management of substance use disorder However, we tried to present information in lay person's language. This book is written in a short story format to visualise how an ordinary person can fall prey to drug and alcohol. What happens to the family of a person using drug and alcohol? Can willpower be enough to curb the desire to drink? Addiction is an illness: believe it or not, and as a society, we need to unite to fight with the monster of addiction.

Dr Gargi Sinha

Table of Contents

Part one 1

Introduction 2

Chapter one 6

Demystifying illness addiction 6

Chapter two 16

Missing elephant in the room... 16

Chapter 3 24

In the shadow of a glass and more 24

Chapter four 29

Sparkling monster hidden in a glittering bottle 29

Chapter five 34

My journey from the shelf of a bottle shop 34

Chapter six 42

Distress call from frontal lobe of brain 42

Chapter Seven 49

Unappreciated endeavour... 49

Chapter 8 57

Cost of crossing the Lakshman Rekha 57

Chapter nine 65

Bird's eye view approach.. 65

Chapter ten 73

Effect of addition on the human body 73

Part two 0

    Addiction Brief Communication Tool 1

    Concept one 3

    When substance use becomes an illness 3

    Concept two 5

    Prevention is better than cure 5

    Concept three 6

    How parent's addiction affects children at home 6

    Concept four 8

    How addiction affect family environment 8

    Concept five 10

    Medical evaluation of addiction 10

    Concept six 11

    Traffic light approach to addiction 11

    Concept seven 14

    Addimeter – a community screening tool for addiction .. 14

    Concept Eight 20

    Cobweb of Addiction 20

Part one

Introduction

Addiction has affected people across the geographical regions. The addictive disorder has a direct effect on a person's physical as well as psychological health. The impact of addiction pervades other aspects of life as well. For instance, it can affect the relationship, family life, social life, education, and employment aspects of life. Unfortunately, we feel embarrassed to talk about addiction. We often minimize the illness addiction and pretends as if everything is normal. While we proudly patronize other chronic medical conditions and glamourize all health professionals associated with their recognition and treatment; however, we stigmatize all professionals providing treatment and care for addictive disorders. Our society generally holds quite a pessimistic view about addiction and tend to believe in the fact that whatever you do, addiction is a personal choice and no intervention can help it. If we take the example of another chronic disease, such as diabetes, which is essentially a progressive disorder irrespective of whatever you do. Patients of diabetes and their family generally express a sense of ownership for their illness and they are generally ready to pay any amount of fees if they have to attend some seminar or education sessions about diabetes. However, substance use disorder is even more destructive than diabetes and it is a 100% treatable condition if treated with proper understanding and support. We usually fail to recognize and treat substance dependence due to failure to persevere hard enough and long enough. It is scientifically proven that substance dependence is a chronic relapsing illness and thus relapse is almost inevitable during the initial period of treatment. The closest situation which can resemble this scenario is eating sweets during initial period of treatment of diabetes. Despite eating sweet foods may shoot up our blood sugar level, but we never stop the medication for diabetes. We never abandon a patient with diabetes for raising their blood sugar due to poor dietary choices. We rather learn from mistakes and try again more strongly to our keep blood sugar level under control. This type of spirit is appallingly missing while we treat a patient of addictive disorder despite, they belong to the same family of chronic diseases.

Unfortunately, we treat the illness addiction as a black sheep in the society and expect an instant and extraordinary outcome from treatment. Our attitude towards a patient with an addictive disorder makes them more ostracized and marginalized in the community. It is beyond doubt that our society needs to change the attitude towards substance use disorder. A persistence and empathic approach are required for long-term success because complete recovery from addiction is inevitable in the long run if we try hard enough and long enough. As King T'Challa rightly said "Wise builds bridges while foolish builds barriers in times of crisis". Thus, we need to build bridges among people and their society to address this complex problem.

The main goal of the book is the empowerment of consumers of substance use disorder. This book has been written in layman's language and illustrated with multiple real-life case scenarios. Some stories have been narrated as direct and first-person conversation of the substance itself with the reader. This book has been written for common people who have limited knowledge about substance use disorder. The names used in the book are fictitious and they have no resemblance to any real-life person. This book will remain a crispy and concise account of the illness addiction, holistic management, and its various psychosocial complications.

Chapter one

Demystifying illness addiction

Where addiction leads to?

Cycle of Disadvantage

Addiction → Loss of job → Financial crisis → Social stigma and exclusion → Poverty and disadvantages transmitted to next generation → Addiction

How does our society view addiction?

Our society views drug addiction with two opposing ideologies: the 'moral' model of addiction and the 'disease' model of addiction. The moral model of addiction entails addiction as a personal choice, and it happens due to moral failure and lack of willpower. In contrast, the disease model of addiction describes an addiction as a disease with a multifactorial origin.

When addiction is considered as a moral problem or character weakness, individuals with addiction problems are subjected to punitive consequences and social stigmatization instead of proper medical treatment for addiction. On the other hand, if addiction is labelled as a medical illness, it bears with it much less stigma and it generally undergoes treatment for the condition. The medical model of addiction identifies this problem with other chronic medical illnesses because the clinical presentation and trajectory of the illness that is influenced by complex interplay of psychological, social, and environmental factors as well as genetic risk.

The proponents of the moral model of addiction blame substance users for their predicament. This is called 'victim-blaming'. Research has shown that victim-blaming is one of the major obstacles for overcoming addiction problem. Blaming the victim attitude of the community often dissuade addicts from seeking help due to embarrassment. The blaming attitude of society helps them to shrug off their responsibility as a member of society. Unfortunately, it produces a culture of denial and ignorance. This attitude produces significant stigma in society about substance use. It is possible to change the culture of victim-blaming by genuinely giving an addict a chance to seek treatment for his or her problem.

How people perceive addiction in real life setting?

Recently, while I was reading a story about the drug menace in India, it reminded me about a real story of my patient in India. This story depicted catastrophic medical consequences due to severe problems with addiction. This story narrated an account of a mother of a son who was afflicted with an addictive disorder. Sita Devi narrated a sad story of her son, Yoginder. He started using drugs when he was still in school. He eventually dropped out of school and befriended with the wrong crowd. During early days, he was addicted to alcohol and then cough syrups and eventually turned into injectable drugs. At one point, Sita Devi recalled, her son wanted to quit and even asked her for help before getting lost into a drug-using lifestyle. Yoginder had no money to support his expensive drug habit. Consequently, Yoginder started selling anything which would come into his sight to buy drugs, Sita Devi said. She felt so helpless whenever her son would become unconscious after taking drugs. After recovering from those unconscious states, he will not remember where he was and what he was doing during the period of unconsciousness. In those moments, Sita Devi would just wish and pray that her son should be better off dead. She would feel guilty for giving birth to this monster son. But now Sita Devi regretted her words.

Because as a mother she always wanted him to lead a normal life, having a family and do some work for his livelihood. But it never happened in her son's life. She wanted to take her son to some drug treatment facilities, but she did not know any facilities nearby where her son could go. One day, when Yoginder became unconscious after injecting some illicit drugs, Sita Devi just took him down to a general hospital, where he was declared brought dead. This tragic story depicts how lack of awareness about substance use problem and its treatment may lead to life threatening consequences.

How much is too much?

Merely using substance does not fulfill the criteria for addiction. Many people use alcohol and other addictive substances for recreation and socialisation. They are only being considered dependent on substance when they display certain criteria, such as intense desire to use substance, difficulties to control its use and continued use despite having significant health and social consequences.

This is the stage when people generally require medical attention.

World Health Organisation strongly supported the medical model of addiction in the International classification of disease (ICD 10). ICD 10 has explicitly documented symptoms of substance dependence, which is identical to other medical illnesses. Cross-cultural research has demonstrated that the symptom pattern of addictive illness is consistently present across the world. Recent research has also reported that there are genetic and peer influence and early childhood adversities making people vulnerable for future addiction.

What does the number crunch suggest?

In 2019, roughly 270 million people (5% of global population aged 15-64 years) reported to using drugs in the previous year. Approximately 35 million people are estimated to suffer from severe substance use disorder, while only 1 in 7 people receive treatment. Vast majority of illicit drugs users were abusing cannabis. People, whoever use opioid, were responsible for two-third of substance related deaths. Approximately 11 million people used injectable drugs, of whom 1.4 million live with HIV and 5.6 million with hepatitis C.

A recent Indian study, which is one of the largest epidemiological study on the pattern of substance use in the world, had recognised the increasing burden of substance use in India. Ministry of social justice and empowerment of India conducted a national household substance use survey from all states and Union Territories. Approximately just over two lakhs households were visited by surveyors in 186 districts. Tripura ranked amongst one of the highest alcohols consuming states. Moreover, the National survey revealed that 16 crores Indians are a current user of drug and alcohol. One in five of these consumers is a dependent user and requires urgent treatment. The survey had also identified that there was a major gap in the availability of treatment services in India, only 1 in 200 for alcoholics and 1 in 29 for illicit drug users receives treatment.

Additionally, the survey suggested that one in every seven Indians is an alcohol consumer, making alcohol the most used addictive substance in the country followed by cannabis, opioids, sedatives, and inhalants. Approximately 10 crores of Indians were current users of alcohol and around 5.7 crores of them are estimated to be dependent on alcohol. Roughly two crores of the Indian population were cannabis user with Punjab and UP remains the highest using states. Just under 1 crore abused pharmaceutical opioids, such as codeine cough syrup, opioid pain medications etc. and an almost equal number of populations abused sleeping pills. Inhalational drugs, such as dendrite sniffing were predominantly used by children and adolescents, 4 lakh children use inhalational drugs. Inhalants are the only category of substances for which the prevalence of current use among children and adolescents is higher (1.17%) than adults (0.58%). Nationally, it is estimated that there is about 8.5 Lakh injecting illicit drugs and injectable drug use is widely prevalent in the North-eastern of states of India. All injectable drug users are at higher risk of contracting HIV and hepatitis C due to unsafe needle practices.

In terms of access to treatment services, the current situation in India paints an appalling picture as well. Approximately 1 in 38 people with alcohol dependence reported getting any treatment. Only about 1 in 180 people with alcohol dependence reported getting inpatient treatment/hospitalization for help with alcohol problems. Among people suffering from dependence on illicit drugs, one among 20 people had ever received inpatient treatment/ hospitalization for help with drug problems.

This national survey strongly supports the severity and extent of problem addiction and identified a significant gap in health services to address this problem. Therefore, the illness model of addiction is now well established. Our society should work together to have a paradigm shift towards illness model of substance use disorder, and it should endeavour to utilise the opportunities to treat the condition and complications associated with it.

Chapter two

Missing elephant in the room

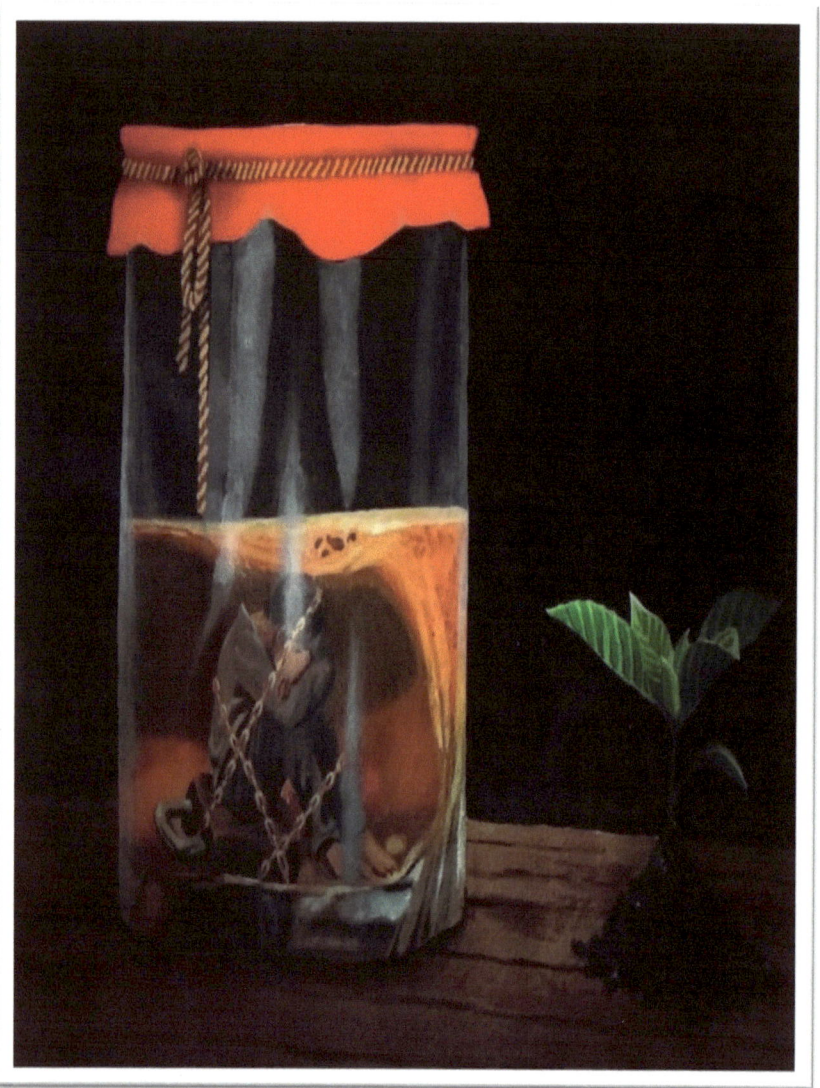

What happens to the children whose parents suffer from addiction?

The impact of addiction often goes beyond the adult member of the family and affect their children. Harmful effect of addiction on children can be prevented by identifying and supporting them from their early childhood. Traditional addiction treatment services often fail to recognize the big elephant in the room, called 'children of addicts.

Laila is a nineteen-year-old girl from far North-Eastern region of India. Laila was born into a low-income family as the eldest child among three siblings. Despite being raised in poverty, she had a happy family until the unwanted' substance secretly crept into her father's life. Her dad, who was working as a labourer, started loving alcohol more than his wife and children. Gradually, her father started spending most of his wages on alcohol while neglecting his family. Her mother had to join a basic housekeeping job to sustain their family. Her mother did not give up hope. She tried to help her husband to overcome his habit of alcohol; however, she failed miserably after multiple attempts. Subsequently, her father started complaining of frequent vomiting and abdominal pain. He was feeling too weak to go to work. His hospital visits became more frequent, and finally, the doctor diagnosed him with pancreatitis. The pancreas is an important organ in our body, which releases enzymes helping with digestion of food. She can still remember tears in her mum's eyes when her father was diagnosed with pancreatitis. Her mother was feeling utterly helpless and tired of arranging money to pay for her husband's medical bills. In absence of her mother at home, Laila had to care of her younger siblings; for instance, cooking meals for them, sending them to school, and looking after them. As a result, she could not perform well in her studies and received bad grades in the class tests. It shattered her confidence and damaged her self-esteem. She started staying at home and withdrew from her friends as she was ashamed of her grades. She didn't know where she could get some help. The society started putting pressure on Laila's mother to get her married at a very young age. She was a young girl with hopes and a twinkle in her eyes like any other girls of her age group. However, alcohol addiction in her father had unfortunately snatched away her dreams and forced her to the cycle of poverty and disadvantage.

What is Second-hand Drinking?

Lisa Frederiksen, a daughter of an alcoholic mom, coined the term 'Second-hand Drinking'(SHD) to refer to the negative impact of alcoholic parents on their children. Approximately 1:3 children of parents with addiction develops substance use disorder, in their adult life, and they are introduced to a substance at a very young age. Living with substance dependent parents can be compared with 'living in the war zone', where family dynamic revolves around chaos and unpredictable behaviour of addicted parents. To avoid confrontation with substance users, family members often pretend that everything is normal in their home. This causes a serious psychological impact especially to the vulnerable members of the family, such as children. They experience significant shame and guilt but remain either in denial or being a silent spectator. However, they are generally not allowed to share their family secret with others. Thus, children learn to live with psychological pain by repressing it into their unconscious mind.

What emotional cost children pay?

As research has suggested that children's early experiences with the parents make the foundation of their future behaviour and determine how they are going to relate to others. In the absence of this foundation, children develop a fragile self-image, which makes them vulnerable to major mental health problems in future, such as depression, anxiety, and substance use problem. Additionally, children may develop post-traumatic stress disorder after witnessing frequent domestic violence between their parents. They frequently make wrong choices about their life partner in future. They miss out in studies and usually get deviated from their career trajectory. Their life gets halted in a stage, when children with normal upbringing endeavour to develop their personality, learn social skill, and build up a sense of trust within themselves. As a result, 'children of addicts' find it hard to fit into normal society. They become socially isolated and often resort to substance abuse to cope with their sense of isolation.

What is parentification?

Another phenomenon observed in 'children of addicts' when they become parent of their parents. Adults, who suffer from substance dependence, are usually unable to perform their duties and family responsibilities. Once a child takes responsibility for their addict parents, they suffer from terrible consequences. They often do it at the expense of their own developmental needs. This is called 'Parentification', which was coined by Boszormenyi-Nagy and Spark. Parentification compromises needs of children. For instance, children of parents with serious addiction problem are forced to grow up quickly often at the cost of their own needs. The process of parentification poses an enormous risk to children which can go beyond their school life. Parentification poses a serious threat to child's psychological health and emotional development during critical period of their life, having a long-term ramification in in development of their identity, self-esteem, and personality.

Despite that, there are only limited services available in the community, which specifically look at the impact of substance dependence on the vulnerable children. Additionally, our education system is not sensitive enough to detect and nurture this group of traumatised little souls. Thus, early detection and welfare of children of addicts is the need of the hour because this will not only help them to stay on the track but also prevent the downward spiral in their later life.

Chapter 3

In the shadow of a glass and more

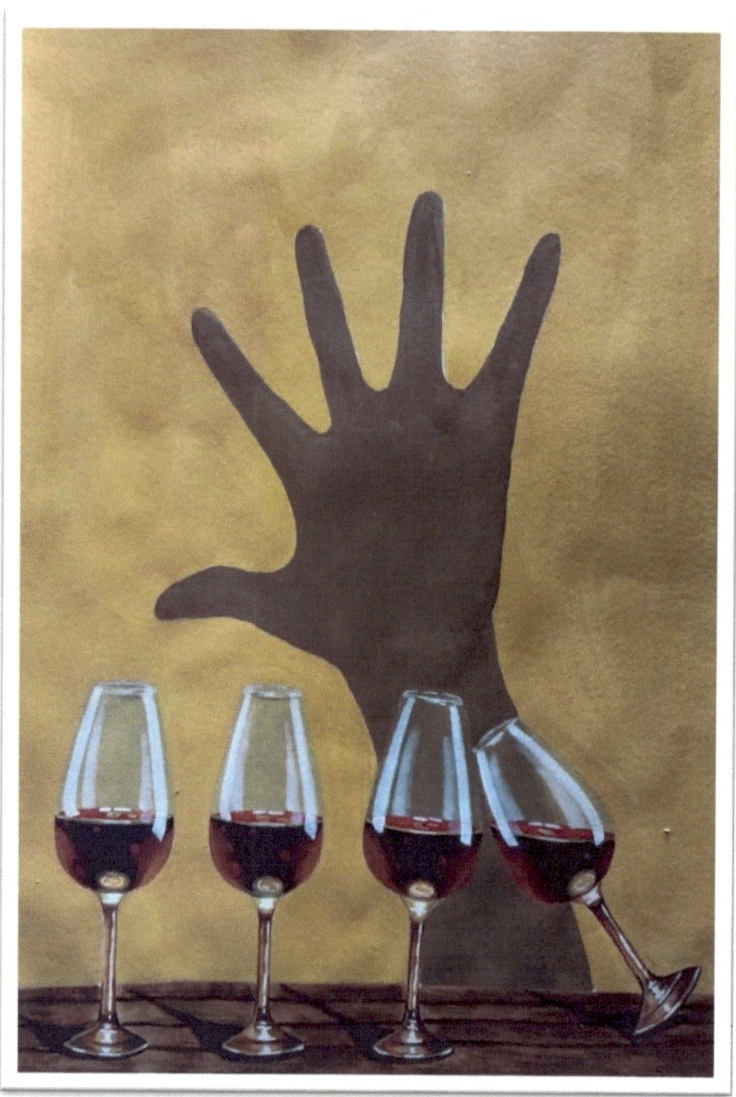

Why talking about addiction at an early young age is necessary?

Adolescence age is a critical period of development of human life. Adolescence is the period of life when children endeavour to achieve life skills, develop their self-identity and personality. Thus, any disruption in this phase of life cycle, such as substance abuse can affect entire trajectory of life.

An anonymous university student narrated a short story about how his life thrown into a downward spiral due to alcohol dependence. It all started with the habit of having one or two glasses of wine during his college days. His life in young age was full of fun. He had a large network of friends. He was feeling proud to secure his first job immediately after completion his graduation. His life was a blessing for him as it was moving in the right direction. However, stress at work started to build up slowly. Work stress made him so overwhelmed that he began to drink a glass or two of wine to cope with stress. Gradually, his behaviour had changed. He became quite impulsive, and aggressive after an episode of drinking. His drinking habit further escalated; he would frequently go to his office under influence of alcohol. He met an accident while drunk driving, and after being breath analysed, police found his blood alcohol level approximately three times above the legal limit. Despite repeated warnings, he could not resist the urge to drink at his office. Eventually, he lost his job. One or two glass of wine was no longer enough for him and his level of alcohol consumption rose astronomically. Excessive drinking of alcohol resulted in new health problems for him. Accidents became more frequent. He started to experience abdominal pain. Some even noticed that he was forgetting things which was out of character. Gradually, his appearance became much older than the buddies of his age group, but still, his attraction for a glass of wine did not dissipate; he rather attributed his poor eating habit to his physical health problems. He often skipped his meals to drink more glasses of wine and he would also forget to eat his regular meals after drinking. When everything progressed too far, he would regret for his mistake for not saying no to his first glass of wine. He wished if he could go back to his younger age and stop at the first glass of alcohol, perhaps he would never spend the rest of his life in the shadow of glass and more. This story reveals the fact that substance use disorder is a progressive medical illness, which has resemblance to other chronic medical illnesses, such as diabetes. If it can be intervened at the younger age, the extent of negative effects of addiction can be minimised as prevention is always better than cure.

Chapter four

Sparkling monster hidden in a glittering bottle

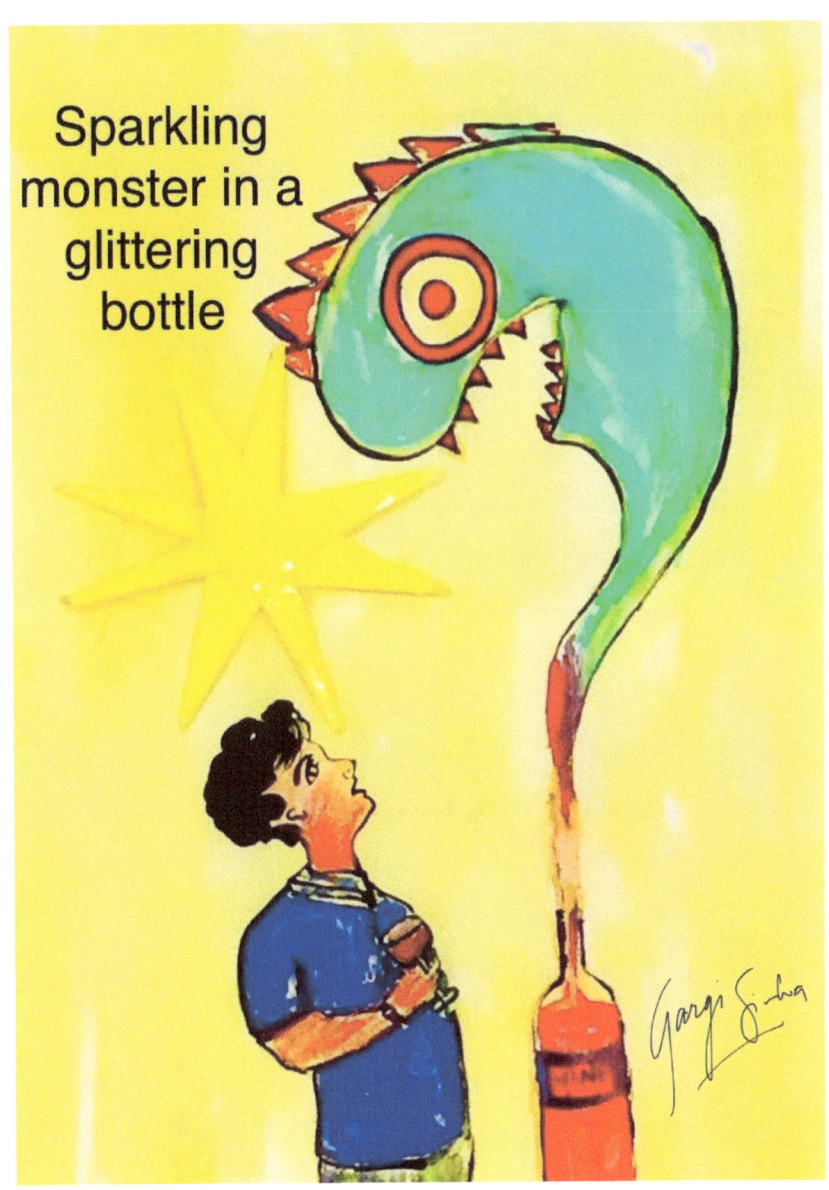

How young people trapped in cycle of addiction?

The journey of addiction usually starts from teenage years. As adolescence transitions to young adult age, a glittering bottle in the shop or restaurant often attracts them. Despite hearing scary stories about the monster captured in the shiny bottle, however, young people still get tempted to pour the beast in a glass or two. When they drip these ripples in the glass, the colour, and the texture of it becomes quite alluring to them. By holding a beer mug or wine glass in hand, a youth rejoice the power of transitioning to adulthood.

As time progresses, young people slowly fall in love with the shimmering bottle while discounting the negative effect of drinking alcohol. Although, alcohol in the bottle is colourful, relaxing, and attractive; however, it is, after all, a monster which is trapped inside a closed lid of a transparent container and waiting to reveal its true monster power to the individual using it, which is often extended to the family and the wider community. The domino effect of alcohol slowly knocks down all assets of a person's like blocks of domino, and soothing and relaxing ripples of the colourful liquid is completely surpassed by harmful side of it.

When a youth is afflicted with substance dependence enters their midlife, their bank balance is mostly spent on the extra bottle or two of alcohol. Their friends often abandon them, and their family members disown them due to their daily drama of violence and disruption at home under influence of alcohol. Additionally, they struggle to sustain their work due to frequent hangovers. Thus, the monster in the bottle destroys whole life of a person.

Fortunately, the monster can be tamed if intervened at the early age. Before opening the glittering bottle, young people should remember that they are pouring a sparking monster in the glass, which is a deadly monster, even though it looks quite alluring inside the transparent glass bottle. The monster, which does not differentiate between rich or poor, uneducated, or educated, and it relentlessly destroys the health of the person, his family life and social life. Therefore, awareness and support at early age can prevent devastating consequences of substance dependence at young age.

Domino Effect of Substance Dependence

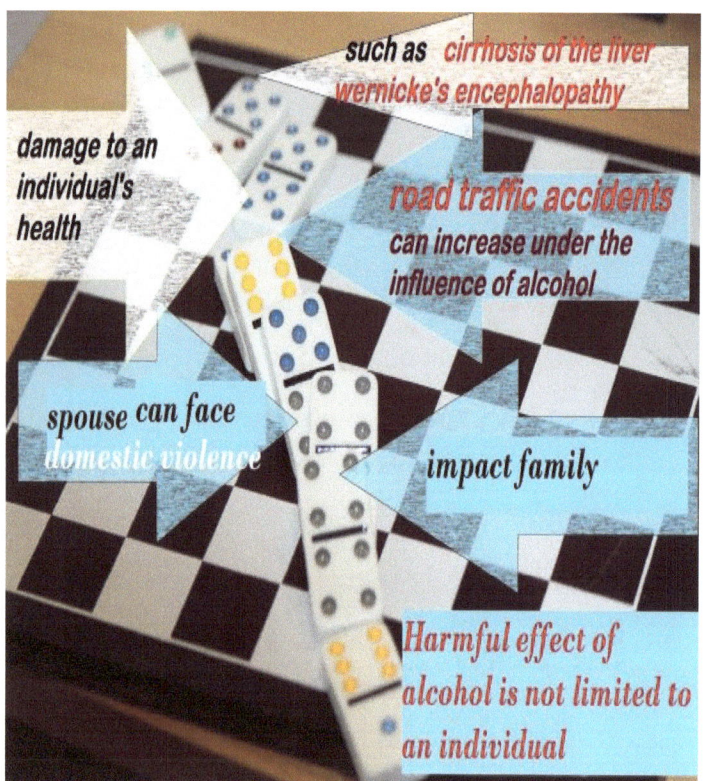

Chapter five

My journey from the shelf of a bottle shop

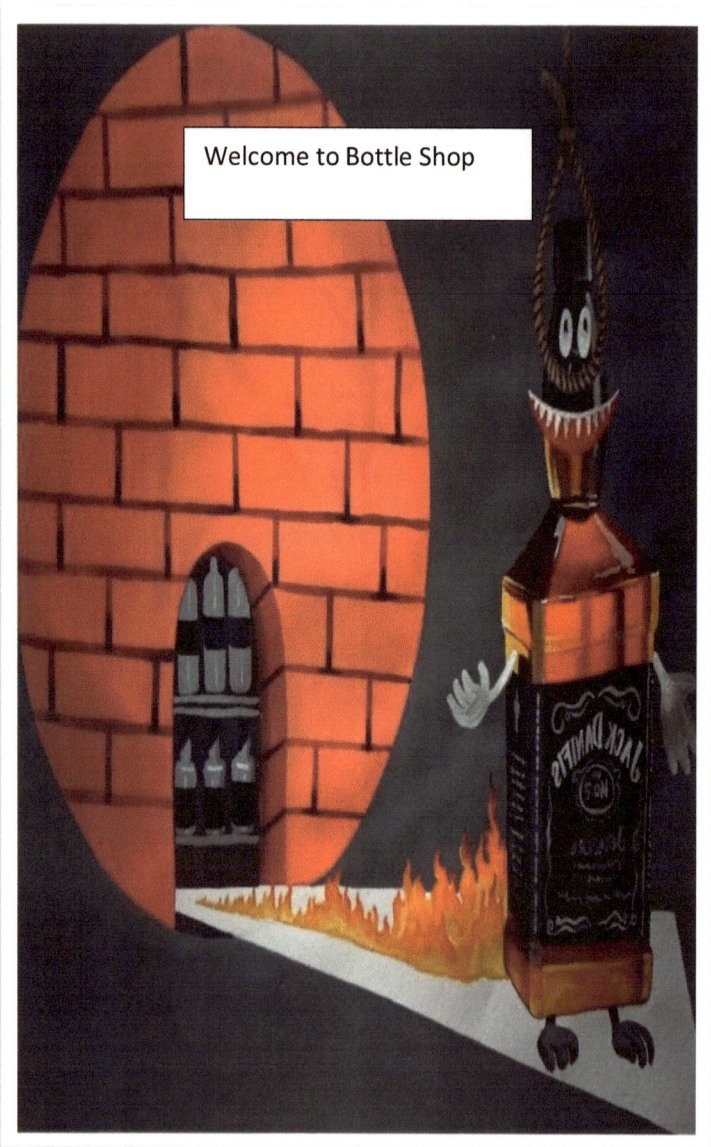

What a bottle witness sitting on a shelf of a bottle shop?

Many people use substance for recreational reasons in the social situation. Recreational use of substance may not a problem. However, substance use becomes a matter of concern when people use it regularly, and when they experience significant physical and psychological harm due to the ongoing use of substance. Substance withdrawal symptoms are cluster of symptoms which emerge when someone decides to suddenly stop using substance after a period of regular use. The journey of alcohol starts from the bottle shop and leads to a devastating consequence on the human body.

Once I was silently sitting on the shelf of a bottle shop and waiting for my turn to be picked up by some admirer of mine. I waited for a month until a twenty-year-old man came to the shop. Desperately, the young man picked me up and went to the counter to pay the bill and rushed outside to open me. He was sweating and shivering, and I knew he was craving for me right then. "Stop" shouted the superego of the boy. "You haven't touched the bottle for the last 48 hours, then why are you rushing to buy alcohol so urgently?" I chuckled sensing the perplexity of his mind which conflicted with his body. The dilemma inside his mind completely paralysed him as his brain was craving for alcohol whereas his body was feeling exhausted. Despite his all efforts to stay sober, craving overpowered him, and he started gulping me quickly to calm his nerves down. He became intoxicated instantly. His brain cells began to slow down. He became quite wobbly on his feet and suddenly fell on the ground.

The young man tried to get up from the ground, but he could not, and then he aggressively started yelling at strangers on the street. Soon after, police arrived and asked him to stand up. He was still unsteady on his feet and was struggling to walk. After all, he needed to go to the police station for displaying antisocial behaviour in the public place.

When people pour me in the glass, they rarely realise how can I damage their career, family, health, and reputation. Even though I am a legal substance, but it does not mean that I am harmless. Perhaps, my glossy labels and bright colour create an illusion of being harmless. Despite looking sparkling and colourful from my external appearance, I am addictive to an individual, destructive to their family and catastrophic for their community.

Why people are so desperate to pick a bottle?

Substance use disorder usually leads to a downhill course in the human body. It slowly destroys physical health, mental health, and quality of life. The substance, which usually starts as a mean for recreation, gradually jeopardises almost all areas of human life. With ongoing use of a substance, brain cells become increasingly dependent on it. Thus, people need more and more substance to have the same buzz. If they miss even a single dose of a substance, they experience terrible withdrawal symptoms. Withdrawal symptoms can only be relieved by using substance again. As a result, a vicious cycle is set up. Eventually, substance becomes so entrenched in their life that their willpower is not enough to overcome it. Medical treatment alone cannot also bring the desired change in the substance using individual. To curb the storm created by substance use, a coordinated approach from the individual, family and the community is required.

Is it possible to get out of bottle craving?

Early detection and treatment can ameliorate harm associated with substance use. The most common deterrents for treatment of addiction is withdrawal symptoms and craving (compelling desire to use substance). Withdrawal symptoms can be quite overwhelming, and it always compel people to use substance again despite having negative consequences. Both withdrawal symptoms and carving can be successfully treated with medications and behavioural intervention. Community and healthcare providers can educate problematic substance users about short-term nature of withdrawal symptoms, which can be treated with medication. Additionally, psychological treatment, such as brief intervention or motivational counselling can help to reduce amount of substance use and high-risk behaviours associated with substance use, such as driving under influence.

Brief intervention is a short 5-15 minutes targeted counselling session which has shown to reduce alcohol drinking in non-dependent drinkers or recreational substance users. Any person with limited experience for the treatment of substance use disorder can conduct a brief intervention session if they have some basic training about it. The 'FLAGS' of brief intervention are as following:

Feedback- Provide individual feedback about the harm already caused by the substance in them and risks of future damage to physical and psychological health from continuing use of substance. For instance, poor sleep, lack of energy, memory problems, weight loss, high blood pressure and injury to internal organs.

Listen- Actively listen to the patient and put their exact verbatim in the context during reflective discussion.

Advice- Provide concise and non-judgemental information on pros and cons of substance use. Some benefits of cutting down drinking, such as better sleep, more energy level, no hangover, better memory, improvement of concentration, improvement of mood, saving money and improving physical health parameters. All these benefits need to be weighed up against cons of staying sober in a non-confrontational environment.

Goals- Encourage the patient to set a specific time-bound goal of their daily consumption of alcohol based on safe drinking guideline.

Strategies- Encourage the patient to develop some plans to achieve the goals. Some examples include drink only with solid food, drink a glass of water in between drinks, switching to smaller glass size, consuming low alcohol content drink, avoiding to drive after drinking, keeping a small amount of pocket money and designating a specific time and place for drinking. Developing some alternative pleasurable activities or coping strategies may minimise tendency to drink when feeling bored and stressed out.

Chapter six

Distress call from frontal lobe of brain

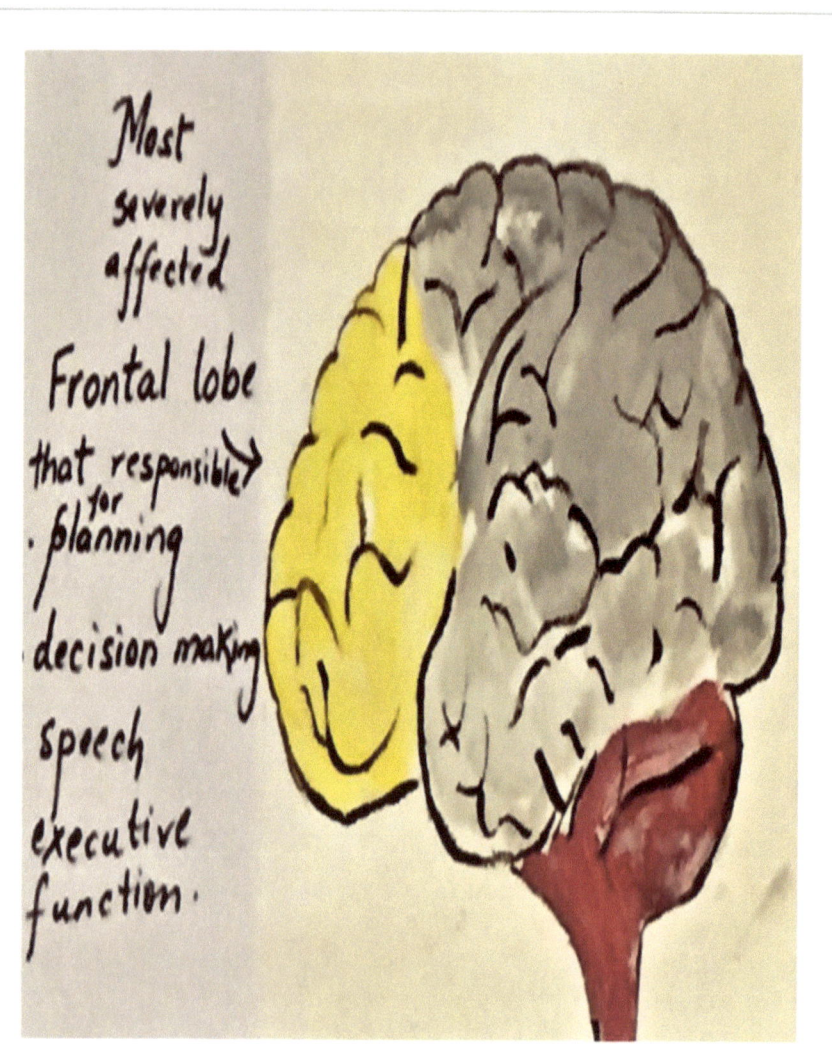

What is frontal lobe?

The frontal lobe is an important part of the human brain. Human beings are different from all other living creatures due to frontal lobe. The frontal lobe can be considered as our brain's 'think tank'. Frontal lobe is a special gift for human beings in comparison to other living organisms. Frontal lobe is responsible for the executive function of our brain. It plays several important roles in our day to day life. The frontal lobe is also responsible for planning and decision making. Frontal lobe controls emotional responses and organisational skill as well. It also takes part in memory function and speech. Research has proven that ongoing substance use can put frontal lobe under incredible strain.

A letter from frontal lobe

Hi Mr/Mrs XY,

I am your frontal lobe of the brain. I feel annoyed while discussing about my predicament. Perhaps my current terrible condition is no way depicting the past glorious time I had spent with you. During your childhood, I can recall that you were academically brilliant and always made your parents proud due to your academic achievement and your modest behaviour. Still, I can vividly recall those days when your intelligence and personality would attract everyone's attention. That was because I was fully functioning on those days and was always being able to invigorate intelligence and calmness. I can also recall the phase of your life when you started drinking alcohol for social lubrication, to overcome stress and a sense of loneliness. Back then, you were probably quite naive to appreciate that occasional alcohol drinking may even cause some harm to you. But I must admit here that it was becoming quite uncomfortable for me to cope with your increasing consumption of alcohol as alcohol was certainly slowing me down. Can you remember the night when I was trying to send a signal to the foot to slow down your car, but you disregarded me, and crashed into another car? It was a horrible night, wasn't it? After the accident, you had to deal with hospital, police and court, all messes in one night. Perhaps, I cannot remember everything now. I am so fragile now that I cannot even help you with making plans about your daily affairs. Recently, I have noticed that you have been making impulsive and hasty decisions. I have also realised that I have been gradually losing my control over your personality, emotion, and behaviour.

Despite that, you kept on dissolving me in gallons of alcohol. I do understand it was not your fault as your body is biologically dependent on alcohol, and your tolerance has increased by several folds. I was not aware at that time, what the term 'tolerance' means. Gradually I have recognised that you were requiring the same substance at the higher quantity to get the same effect. I cannot blame you because I started dissolving by then and I could not make you aware of the changes that have occurred to you.

I won't say that you never tried to give up, you sincerely tried to get rid of alcohol on several occasions. But I hated the withdrawal symptoms from alcohol, which made everything so difficult to conquer. I disliked the shakes of the body, weakness, feeling sick and vomiting after abstinence from alcohol for a day or two. Strong shakes after withdrawal from alcohol were feeling like the earthquake to me which would resolve only after alcohol consumption. I can still remember the day when you became unconscious and having convulsions.

Now looking back, I can appreciate that life could have been a blessing if you did not infuse the first drop of alcohol into me. Now I have been crushed and turned into a shrinking piece sitting like wreckage in your skull. I was helplessly observing how you have lost your fame, fortune, and family for a monster whose favourite food is frontal lobe nuggets with liver chips and heart dips.

Yours truly

Frontal Lobe

Save the frontal lobe

Frontal lobe changes can be reversed if intervened early in the course of illness. Frontal lobe damage can completely alter someone's personality. Frontal lobe damage can also cause significant problems with behaviour impacting relationship, work, and studies as well. Good nutrition and total abstinence from addictive substance is the only remedy to reverse the downward spiral of the frontal lobe.

Chapter Seven

Unappreciated endeavour

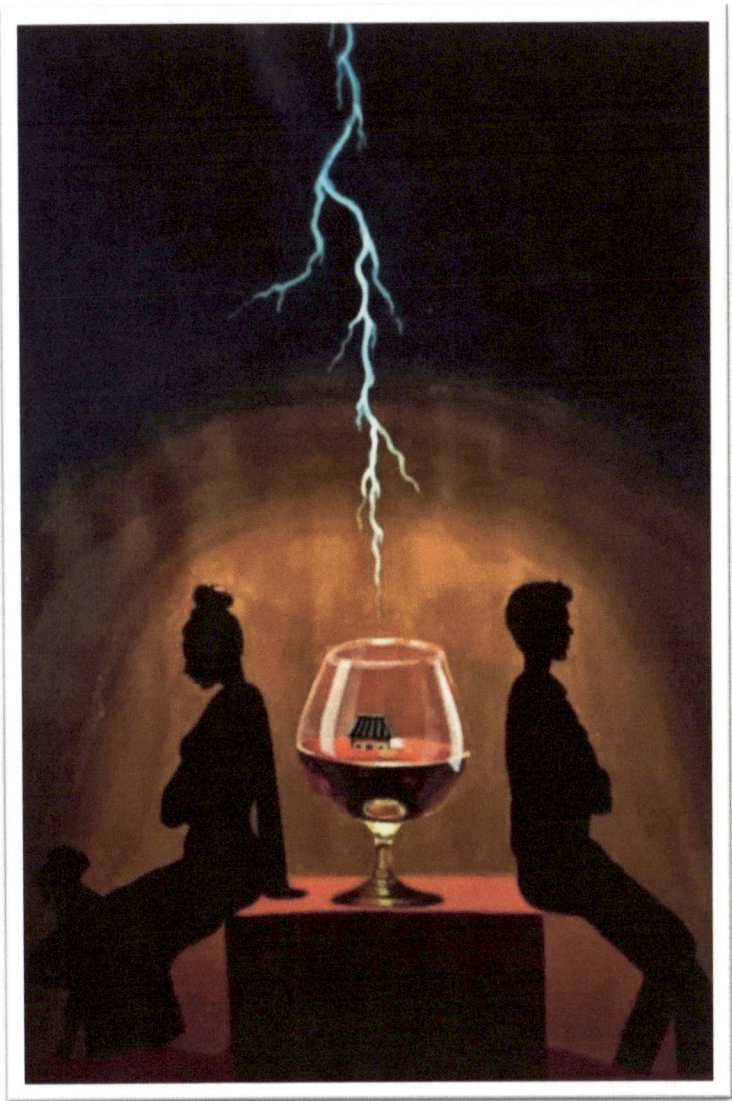

What are the expectations from a wife of people who consume excessive alcohol?

Our society generally hold a high expectation from the wives of substance-dependent persons. Their wives' role is not only restricted to raising their children. They are often forced to become the breadwinner of the family. They are often subjected to horrific domestic violence experiences from their intoxicated partners. They are frequently compelled to visit hospitals to seek treatment for their partners due to different substance-related health complications. Despite their incredible efforts, they frequently become a subject of criticism from society. They are stigmatised and marginalised due to their association with a substance dependent individual. The following story has been drawn from real-life experience of wife of a substance-dependent person. The story has tried to give an overview of life circumstances of the partner a substance using partner and depicted the extent of their suffering from consequences of something which is not their fault.

How illness addiction presents in a community setting?

Once I met a woman in her early twenties at a local vegetable market in a small town in Tripura, India. As we had never met before, she spoke hesitantly, in a feeble voice, saying, "I need to discuss some personal issues with you and need some advice from you." Such instances of village women approaching me were not unusual as no other female doctor was available in the community. However, in this case, I could sense her stress from her facial expression. I assured her that I would meet her in the evening at my home. She came and started telling me about her marital journey, which had begun when she was just 18 years old and explained that she had lost her five years of marital bliss to excessive alcohol consumption by her husband. Her affable husband had gradually become dependent on alcohol, and while he was under the influence of alcohol, there was an increase in verbal abuse and physical violence. Despite all domestic abuse, she wanted to help her husband to get out of the excessive drinking pattern. She was keen to know why her normally well-behaved husband started having memory problems and aggressive behaviour. Above all, she wanted to know what she needs to do to bring him back into the mainstream. Many people who are chronic drinkers are not aware of the neurotoxic effect of alcohol. As a result, they are unaware of the consequences of long-term heavy drinking on their behaviour and the impact of alcohol on their family members. It is unfortunate that alcohol is consumed by the man in the house, and our society leaves women in the house to face the challenge of verbal and physical violence alone in the name of a dysfunctional marriage.

How slowly addiction impact family dynamics

The addiction recovery process is a challenging proposition for the spouses. She often has to deal with their substance using partner on their own. Their emotional roller coaster continues due to relapsing nature of illness. Addictive disorder poses significant trauma to the family members, particularly the spouse. The spouse of the substance dependent partner often has to change their role from being a rescuer of their partner and a helpless and disillusioned family member. The spouse of an addict feels incredible shame and a sense of helplessness due to their inability to break the cycle of addiction despite numerous attempts to do so.

Drug and alcohol addiction often have devastating effects on relationships. It quickly breaks down trust and communication between partners. In many instances the spouse may unknowingly become an enabler by indirectly reinforcing addictive behaviour. It is essential to create a boundary between supportive and enabling behaviour. Additionally, a spouse can send the wrong message to the partner by silently approving their partner's drug dependency. The strict boundary usually sends a strong message to the addicted partners, which indirectly helps them to reflect upon their behaviour and bounce back from rock bottom. It can be overwhelming to set boundaries and discussing with the partners how their drug use is hurting them. However, at times, this is the only way to break the cycle of co-dependency. The spouse of an addict does not need to wait for their partner's willingness to address their addiction problem, but they can lead the way by calling for help. By doing so spouses can send a strong message to their addicted partner that they are no longer partners in their addiction; the addiction, but they still love them as a person. In this way, a bond is formed in the face of winning against the menace together, which empowers a family unit to beat future setbacks.

Similarly, substance dependence has a devastating effect on their parents as well. Parents find it incredibly difficult to see their children going down the spiral due to addiction. When a child is young, they are under the supervision of their parents. When they grow up as an adult, parents do not have that control, but they still have parental worries and a sense of responsibility for them. Parents feel enormous shame and stigma about their children's addiction. Rather than seeking help, parents end up pushing their children away. Parents need to compartmentalise their child from addiction. They need to express their love and support towards their children, but addiction needs their strong disapproval. Parents of addicts often fall into the trap of overprotecting their children, hoping that they will change their behaviour. As a result, parents unknowingly end up in enabling their children's addictive behaviour and they do not allow them to learn from their past mistakes. Therefore, the addiction monster grows bigger in their children.

Where from here?

There are a large body of evidence to suggest that substance dependence has significant impact on their family members. Despite that, family members helplessly bear the brunt of addiction, while our society and government seldom think about their plight in the journey of addiction. Family members of addicts also need necessary support from the community and services to rebuild their lives.

Chapter 8

Cost of crossing the Lakshman Rekha

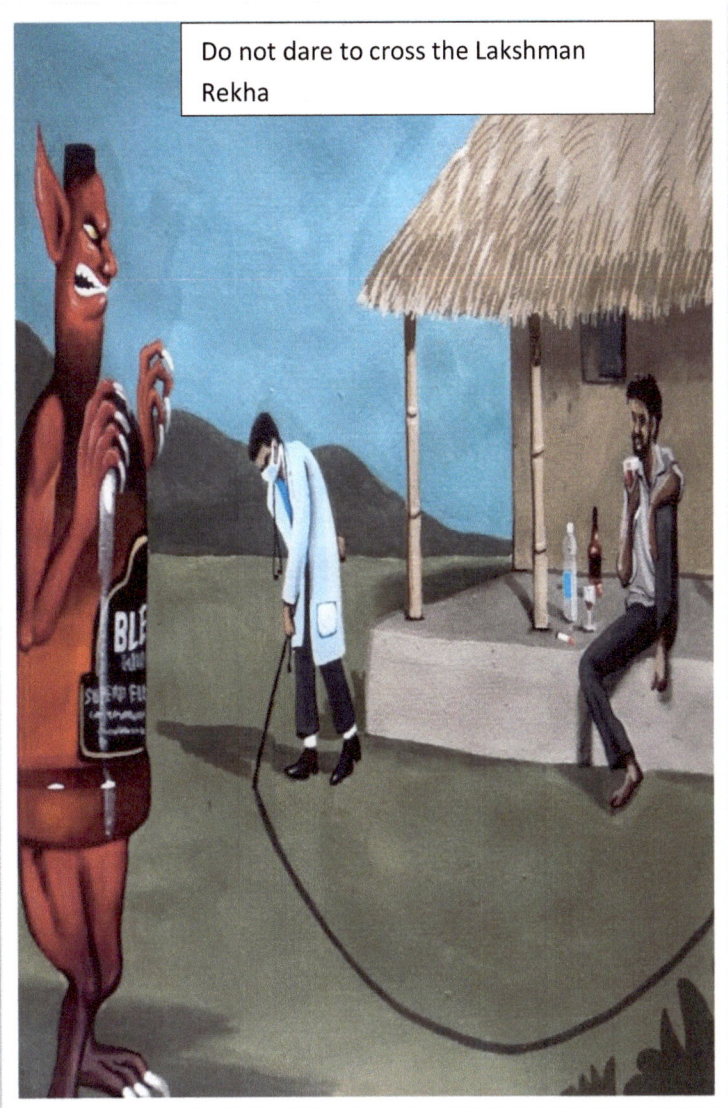

Overview of context Lakshman Rekha

The 'Lakshman Rekha' is a term originally derived from the epic 'Ramayana'. This means a line of demarcation between good and evil or safety and danger. If any situation crosses the Lakshman Rekha, it goes out of control. If we use this concept in the context of substance misuse, it means drawing a line between safe and unacceptable level of substance use. If degree of substance use crosses the Lakshman Rekha, people are expected to experience a wide range of physical and psycho-social complications from substance. In this situation, people usually feel quite helpless and disempowered, and they often require some external help to recover from substance use.

In the story, Princess Sita was kidnapped by 'Ravan' who used to be a tyrannic and powerful king of Lanka Kingdom. Once Ravan was roaming around in his flying chariot, he saw Sita residing in a small cottage in the forest. Sita was living there with her husband Lord Rama and brother in law Lakshman. They started living there after being exiled from their Kingdom Ajodhya following some family conspiracy. Ravan was mesmerised with the elegant beauty of princess Sita. He decided to elope with her and then marry her. Ravan planned to trick her. Ravan changed his appearance to a monk and entered the premises of Sita's house while asking for some alms. Lakshman was concerned about leaving Sita in the isolated cottage but he had to accompany with his brother Lord Rama to the jungle to collect some valuable thing she demanded from her husband. He drew a line on the ground around the cottage and asked Sita not to step out of the line at any cost. Ravan came to the cottage in disguise and was pleading for help. Sita, being a kind-hearted lady, could not resist her temptation to step out of the Lakshman Rekha to offer some alms to the poor monk, who was unfortunately Ravan in disguise. Ravan took this opportunity to capture Sita and dragged her into his Chariot and then he flew away with her back to his gigantic palace in the kingdom of Lanka. Ravan put Sita in a highly secure zone of the palace called Ashok Vatika. Once Ravan went to meet Sita and offered her to get married to him. When Sita refused his proposal straight away, he got furious and told her that no one would be able to reach her in the secluded place. Thus, she should better off change her mind and marry him. Despite the catastrophe, Sita mumbled optimistically that Sri Ram will find her soon and set her free from this wicked world. Sita knew at that time that she was helpless, and she waited patiently for help from an outside source. The story of Sita's isolation in Ashok Vatika has some resemblance with the story of people who are trapped in the web of addiction.

People, who are dependent on substance, often downplay the consequences of crossing the limit of safe level of use. Once their brain cells become accustomed to substance for their daily functioning, it becomes quite difficult to overcome the habit. Consequently, people become a prisoner of the substance. They feel quite helpless to stop using substance. As a result, people lose their confidence and they unwillingly surrender their life to the demons of addiction. As it was described in the epic Ramayana that

God Hanuman finally initiated the rescue process of Sita from the custody of Ravan. Similarly, people who suffer from enduring addiction problem require some external help to overcome the hurdles of addiction.

Outside assistance is needed to conquer the demon of addiction. External Support consists of medical management, family support and community involvement. Contrary to the popular belief, medication only strategy generally remains unsuccessful to treat substance dependence and every attempt of failed treatment further reinforces the state of helplessness in the substance user and their family members. Thus, treatment of addiction requires a teamwork from a multi-disciplinary team.

What are the Stages of Changes Cycle?

One of the established methods of addiction treatment is called motivational interviewing. This is a special type of counselling which help people to navigate through different stages of motivation for addiction. The Stage of

Change cycle describes how strategic counselling facilitates slow progression of the motivation for substance use through different stages of motivation cycle. The following is a brief outline of the 'Stages of Change (Prochaska and DiClemente).

1. Pre-Contemplative stage– Individuals at this stage do not usually consider changing. Individual often express as 'I enjoy drinking and don't want to change

2. Contemplative stage- Individual at this juncture is aware of the harm of drinking, however ambivalent to change.

3. Preparation stage -Individual at this stage is prepared to act. The individual will often express I am ready to cut down on alcohol. Goal setting strategies are useful at this stage.

4. Action stage- Individual at this stage is engaged in attempts to reduce or stop drinking

5. Maintenance or relapse stage -Individual at this stage successfully change drinking behaviour, however, need strategies for relapse prevention.

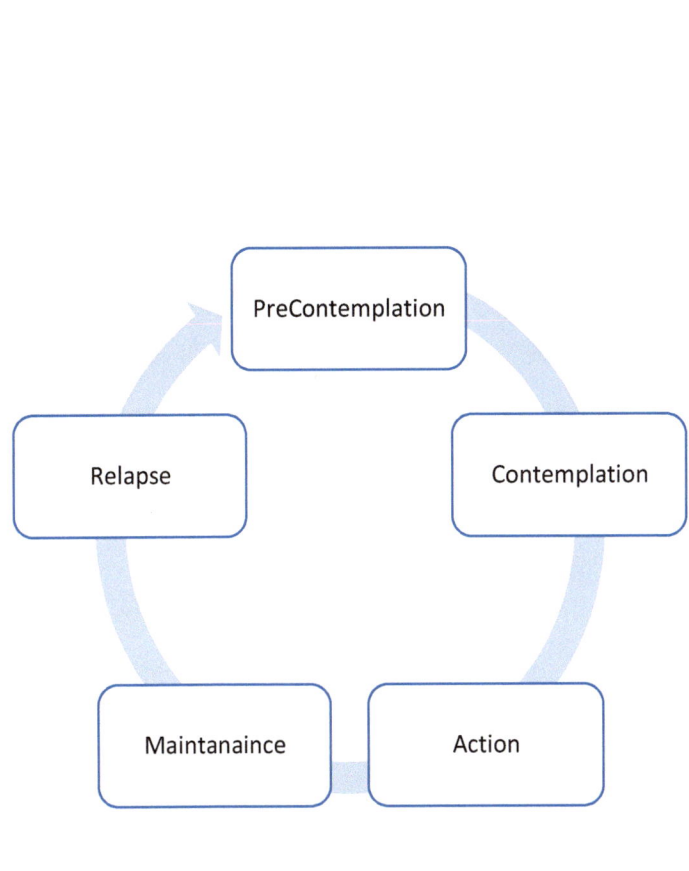

Stages of changes cycle

Chapter nine

Bird's eye view approach

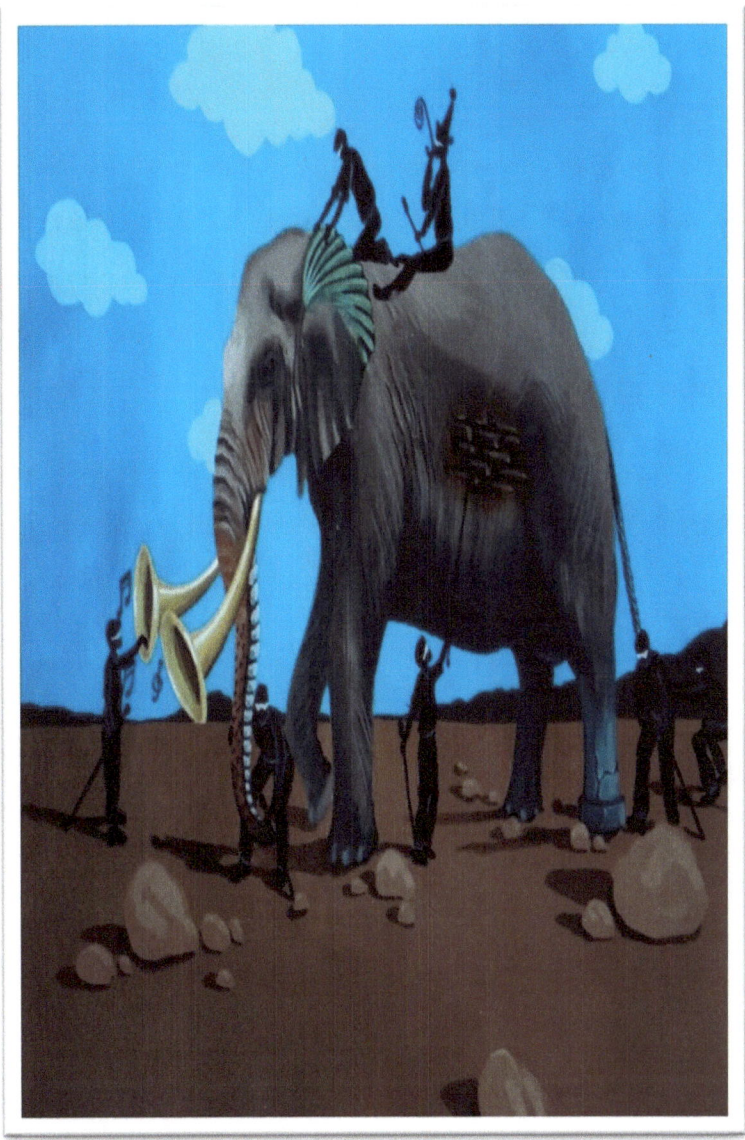

What is bird's eye view?

The bird's eye view literally means viewing from a very high place that allows you to see the whole landscape. It does not focus on one area, but it takes a view of the entire region at a time. In other words, it means a holistic approach.

The parable of six blind men and an elephant depicts how treatment of addiction can have different meaning to different people. Thus, management of substance dependence problem requires a multi-dimensional approach. This story described the experience of a group of blind men when they touched an elephant. Six blindmen were asked to touch an elephant in turns for the first time in their life. Each blindman described their perception of an elephant in their own way. The blind man, who touched the trunk of the elephant, had a different perception in compared to another blind man, who touched the tail of the same elephant. Surprisingly, each of six blind men had a unique view about the appearance of an elephant. An analogy can be drawn between the Six Blind Men story and management of substance use disorder. Our society has a diverse view about the treatment of substance use disorder.

Why do people have diverse opinions about addiction?

While many people may hold an overtly critical view about the treatment of substance use disorder; however, another group of people may consider substance abuse as a chronic relapsing illness requiring ongoing treatment. For instance, many people drink alcohol, but alcohol use is labelled as a medical illness only when it fulfils certain diagnostic criteria, such as withdrawal symptoms, carving, salience, etc. Additionally, there are various stages of motivation for substance use. Thus, the nature of treatment will depend on the motivation of the person. There are many stages of motivation cycle, which was originally proposed by Prochaska and DiClemente in 1983. Since then, their model has become the more popular in the treatment of addiction. This model gives essential insight into patient's stages of behavioural change and their readiness to change their addictive behaviour. The motivation cycle starts with precontemplation, which means total reluctance to change unhealthy behaviour, and the cycle ends with the maintenance stage, which means peoples are motivated enough to sustain their newly learnt sobriety state.

The first stage of addiction treatment is called detoxification or detox. As the name suggests, detox often involves flushing out of the addictive substances from the body. However, medications used for detoxification never flush out toxins, it rather counteracts substance withdrawal symptoms. For instance, diazepam tablet treats alcohol withdrawal symptoms by working on the same area of the brain which is usually being occupied by alcohol. As a result, an alcoholic can easily come off alcohol without suffering much from withdrawal symptoms, such as shakes, lack of sleep, convulsion, and overwhelming anxiety. Different medications are used for different substances. Research has shown that it often requires multiple attempts of detox before maintaining a long-term sobriety state.

Why only medical model of treatment is not enough for illness addiction?

Unfortunately, a vast majority of addiction treatment centres in the world, particularly in developing countries exclusively focus on a detox-based treatment while undermining a more important aspect of addiction treatment. This is called rehabilitation. It is a well-known fact that the effect of addiction goes beyond the index case. Addiction can cause irreparable damage to the family, children, spouse, and society. Additionally, it can cause a significant impact on someone's financial assets and employment opportunities. It drives the entire family unit into the downward spiral of the disadvantage cycle. Furthermore, persons who are inflicted with addiction generally lack the basic life skills and interpersonal skills and they use the substance to mask their underlying deficits. Finally, there is a large body of evidence to suggest that 1 in 2 addicts often suffer underlying mental health problems, such as depression, anxiety, suicidality, etc, which are sadly underdiagnosed and untreated.

Thus, treatment of addiction is more complex than our conventional notion. The famous quote of Albert Einstein is worth mentioning here: 'Everything should be made as simple as possible, but not one bit simpler'. Therefore, offering only detoxication based treatment model, which is a most popular approach for addiction treatment in many countries, will obviously overlook the complex interplay of psychological, social, family, and spiritual factors in the maintenance of the addictive disorder. Success will depend on a coordinated action plan from a team of professionals and substance using peer group. There is some evidence that certain long-term medications can minimise harm by reducing the desire for substance use. However, availability and cost of medication may cause deterrence particularly in low resource settings in the developing countries. Additionally, people generally show a high propensity for relapse to addiction due to chronic and relapsing nature of illness. Any signs of relapse at the early stage generally creates a deep sense of demoralisation and helplessness for the patient as well as their family. This is such an overpowering feeling that people often completely give up any hope of recovery and never try to give it another go. This issue is generally overlooked in most of the addiction treatment facilities. Thus, it is incredibly important to empower the patients with addictive disorder with life skills, sound mental health and social stability. The family and children of addicts also require to be empowered with the basic life skills and community supports. Creating a network of recovering addicts can not only bring new clients into the supportive network but it can also help the recovering addicts from relapsing into substance use again due to mutual support and understanding. Therefore, medication treatment for addiction needs to be supplemented with psycho-social and spiritual support.

Chapter ten

Effect of addition on the human body

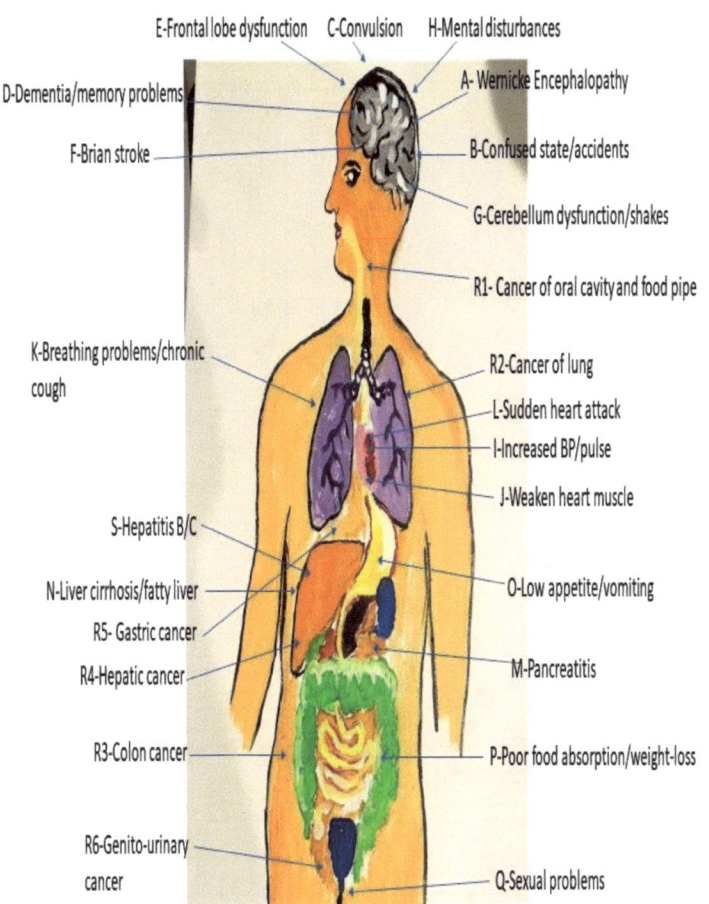

Table represents a human diagram in the previous page. A to S represents wide range of health consequences due to various substance misuse:

	Alcohol	Cannabis	Nicotine	Methamphetamine	Inhalational drugs	Benzodiazepine	Opioid	Cocaine	Hallucinogen
A	■	■			■	■		■	■
B	■			■	■	■		■	
C	■			■	■				
D	■				■				
E	■	■		■				■	
F	■		■	■	■	■		■	
G	■					■	■	■	■
H	■	■		■				■	■
I	■	■	■	■				■	
J	■				■	■	■	■	
K		■	■	■	■		■	■	
L				■					
M	■					■			
N	■						■	■	■
O	■	■		■	■		■		
P	■				■		■	■	
Q	■	■		■	■		■	■	
R	■	■	■	■			■	■	
S				■					

Part two

ABC Tool

Addiction Brief Communication Tool

(For Community Workers and Health Volunteers)

This part of the book is dedicated to practical implementation of knowledge about addiction illness in the grass-root level. Community health workers and volunteers perform an important role in the community in disseminating health education about addiction to the common public. They generally have a limited understanding of addictive disorder and they can comprehend only basic level of language. This part of the book is written in the layman's language and beautifully exemplified by self-explanatory pictures.

Another interesting perspective of this part of book is Addimeter, which is a self-report scale to measure extent and severity of substance use disorder. It takes 5-10minutes to administer. There are seventeen questions in the questionnaire and each item is rated with dichotomous outcomes. The score more than five indicates some problem with substance use and score more than ten indicates severe degree of problem from substance use. At the end, traffic light sign will guide what type of intervention will be required according to the severity of problem.

Concept one
When substance use becomes an illness

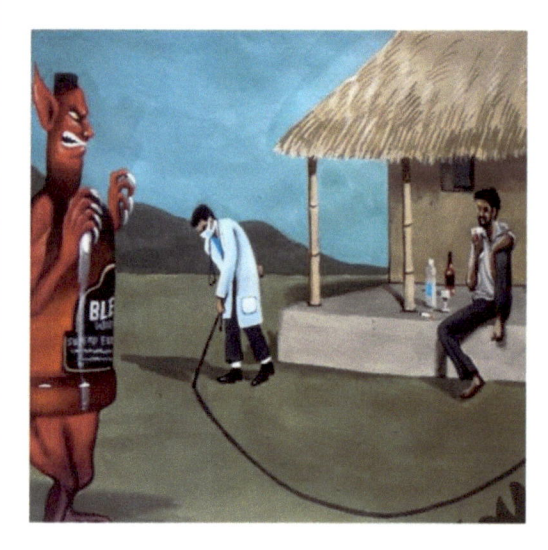

People usually start drinking alcohol in the social situation with their friends, mainly for recreational purposes during their young age. If they continue to drink regularly and heavily, their body gets used to it, and they find it difficult to give up. They become dependent on alcohol for their day to day life functioning. Alcohol dependence is a medical illness. When people cross the 'Lakshman Rekha' of safe and recreation drinking, the monster of addiction destroys their life. There are some certain signs which indicate that people has crossed the safe level of drinking. For example, shaking of hand, lack of sleep without alcohol, feeling sick without alcohol, throwing fits without alcohol, seeing imaginary insects without alcohol and excessive sweating after reducing or stopping alcohol consumption. When they cross the 'Lakshman Rekha' of safe drinking, they experience strong craving after walking up in the morning.

Concept two
Prevention is better than cure

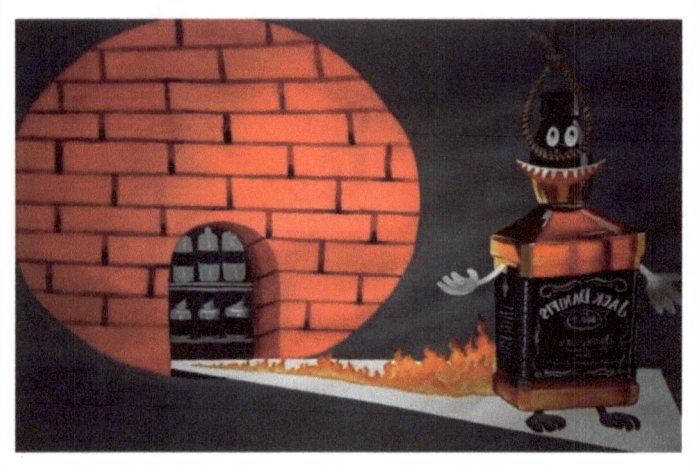

The journey of alcohol starts from a bottle shop. Gradually, it pervades all aspects of human life. It affects our physical health, mental health, social life, family life, employment, and financial resources. An addicted person becomes disconnected from their supportive network and leads a lonely life. If journey of alcohol can be stopped before it goes too far, a human life can be saved.

Concept three
How parent's addiction affects children at home

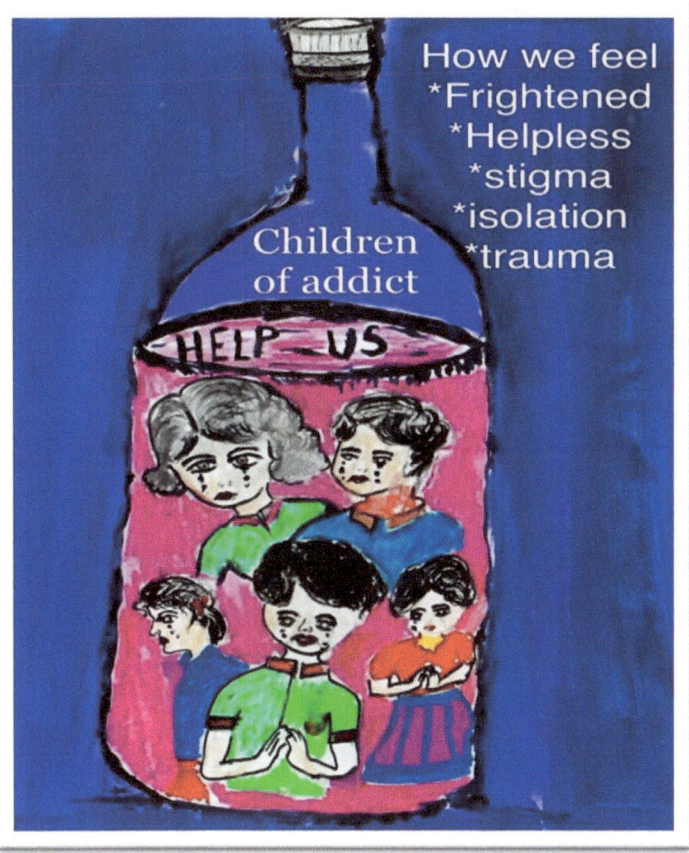

Addiction has a devastating impact on their children. They suffer psychological trauma. They grow up in an environment of fear and uncertainty. They feel ashamed of their parent's addictive behaviour. They feel emotionally neglected by their addicted parents. Children often plays the role of the parent in the family. As a result, their study gets hampered and they disconnect from school and friends. They usually lag their peers and many of them drop out from the school and become an addict themselves. Harmful effect of addiction on children can be prevented by identifying and supporting them from their early childhood. Traditional addiction treatment services often fail to recognize the big elephant in the room, called 'children of addicts.

Concept four
How addiction affect family environment

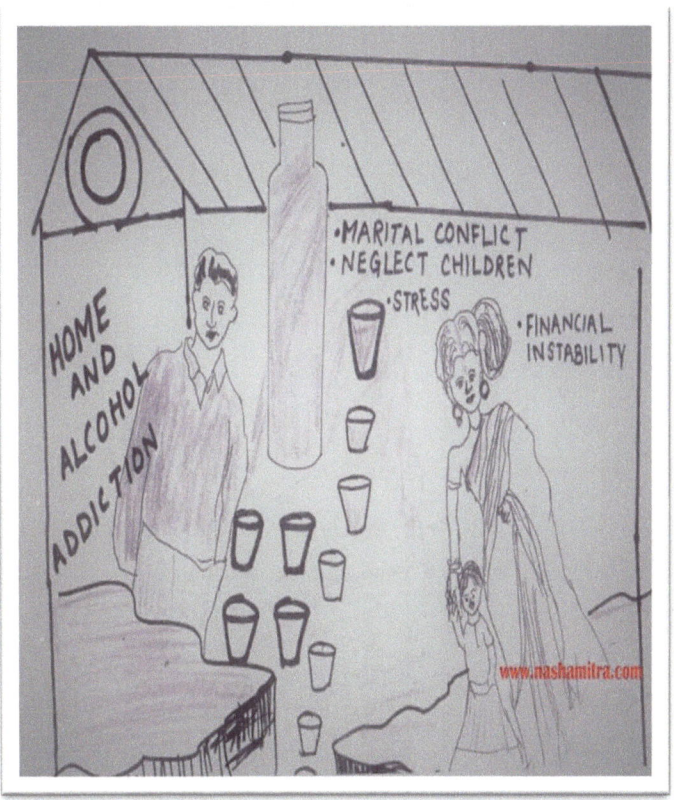

Our society generally hold a high expectation from the wives of substance-dependent persons. Their wives' role is not only restricted to raising their children. They are often forced to become the breadwinner of the family. They are often subjected to horrific domestic violence experiences from their intoxicated partners. They are frequently compelled to visit hospitals to seek treatment for their partners due to different substance-related health complications. Despite their incredible efforts, they frequently become a subject of criticism from society. They are stigmatised and marginalised due to their association with a substance dependent individual. Family members helplessly bear the brunt of addiction, while our society and government seldom think about their plight in the journey of addiction. Family members of addicts also need necessary support from the community and services to rebuild their lives.

Concept five
Medical evaluation of addiction

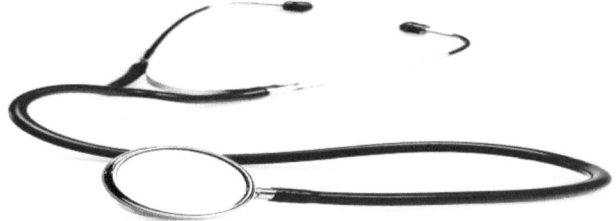

Every person, who is dependent on substance, requires doing a range of medical tests, For example, blood test, tracing of heart (ECG) and whole-body physical examination by a trained physician. They also need to see a psychiatrist or addiction specialist doctor for comprehensive understanding of their problems. An addict dies at least ten years earlier than his same age group people because they often neglect their health despite it is showing obvious signs of stress.

Concept six
Traffic light approach to addiction

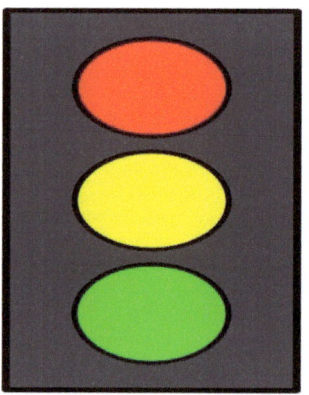

A vast majority of addiction treatment centres in the world, particularly in developing countries exclusively focus on medication-based treatment while undermining a more important aspect of addiction treatment. This is called rehabilitation. Addiction can cause irreparable damage to the family, children, spouse, and society. Additionally, it can cause a significant impact on someone's financial assets and employment opportunities. It drives the entire family unit into the downward spiral of the disadvantage cycle. Furthermore, persons who are inflicted with addiction generally lack the basic life skills and interpersonal skills and they use the substance to mask their underlying deficits. Approximately, 1 in 2 addicts often suffer underlying mental health problems, such as depression, anxiety, suicidality, etc, which are sadly underdiagnosed and untreated. Thus, addicts can be classified into three groups:

Green group are occasional drinker. They usually drink socially with their friends. They are aware of harmful effect and usually drink safely. They do not require any specialised treatment apart from some education about harmful effects of alcohol.

Yellow group is when addiction starts to affect their life. They become more regular drinker. They face some physical health and social consequences as well. Their family members are usually annoyed due to their drinking habit. This group require special type of counselling. They also require doing some medical testing.

Red group is the most severely affected group. It is because addiction starts to take a toll on almost every aspects of their life. For instance, loss of social reputation, unemployment, deterioration of health, and financial crisis. As a result, their family and old friends end up in abandoning them. Despite all untoward outcome, they continue to drink all the time to keep their physical withdrawal symptoms under control. This leads to a downward spiral of addiction. This group usually require more intensive care, called substance rehabilitation under strict treatment protocol.

Concept seven
Addimeter – a community screening tool for addiction

1. Do you use any addictive substances?

    Yes O   No O

2. Have you used any substance almost every day over last three-months period?

    Yes O   No O

Even one tick mark (√) in this table is enough to score '**YES**' in the above question.

Name of the substance	Present (√)
Alcohol	
Cough syrup	
Opium	
Injectable drugs	
Cannabis	
Cocaine	
Amphetamine like substances	
Inhalational substances	
Sleeping pills	
Tobacco	
Heroin	

3. Have you used any substance on weekly basis or weekends over last three- months period?

Yes O   No O

Even one tick mark (√) in this table is enough to score '**YES**' in the above question.

Name of the substance	Present (√)
Alcohol	
Cough syrup	
Opium	
Injectable drugs	
Cannabis	
Cocaine	
Amphetamine like substances	
Inhalational substances	
Sleeping pills	
Tobacco	
Heroin	

4. Have you used any substance at least once monthly over last three- months period?

       Yes O   No O

Even one tick mark (√) in this table is enough to score '**YES**' in the above question.

Name of the substance	Present (√)
Alcohol	
Cough syrup	
Opium	
Injectable drugs	
Cannabis	

Cocaine	
Amphetamine like substances	
Inhalational substances	
Sleeping pills	
Tobacco	
Heroin	

5. Have you ever tried to reduce or stop using any substance over last three-months period?

   Yes O   No O

6. Have experienced **any** physical withdrawal symptoms when you tried to reduce or stop any substance over last three-months period?

   Yes O   No O

Even one tick mark (√) in this table is enough to score '**YES**' in the above question.

Physical withdrawal symptoms	**Present (√)**
Fast heartbeat	
Breathing difficulties	
Sweatiness	
Headaches	
Nausea	
Vomiting	
Diarrhoea	
Running nose	
Dizziness	

Aches and pains	
Convulsions	

7. Have you ever experienced **any** psychological withdrawal symptoms when you tried to reduce or stop any substance over last three-months period?

     Yes O   No O

Even one tick mark (√) in this table is enough to score '**YES**' in the above question.

Psychological withdrawal symptoms	Present (√)
Irritable mood	
Anxiety/tension	
Depression	
Suicidal thoughts	
Lack of sleep	
Aggressive behaviour	
Seeing unusual objects	
Hearing of vices/noises	
Agitation	
Restlessness	
Decreased concentration	
Confusion/disorientation	

8. Have you ever experienced any psychological illnesses due to substance use over last one-year period?

     Yes O   No O

9. Have you ever experienced any legal problems due to substance use over last one-year period?

Yes O   No O

10. Have you ever had any financial difficulties due to substance use over last one-year period?

    Yes O   No O

11. Have you ever experienced any physical health problems due to substance use over last one-year period?

    Yes O   No O

12. Have you ever tried to cut down or stop using any substance due to substance related complications over last one-year period?

    Yes O   No O

13. Have you ever experienced any problems at work due substance use over last three-months period?

    Yes O   No O

14. Have you ever failed to do your daily chores or daily duties due to substance use over last three-months period?

    Yes O   No O

15. Have you ever felt guilty about your substance use over last one-year period?

    Yes O   No O

16. Has your family member or friend expressed concerns about your substance use over last one-year-period?

Yes O   No O

17. Have you ever seen any doctor for substance related problems over last one-year period?

Yes O   No O

Answer to all questions are scored except question number 5 which does not carry any score. If score is more ≥ 5, there is a high likelihood that substance use is a problem and need some medical attention.

Total Score -

Severe – score 11-16. They must seek help of a specialist addiction services.

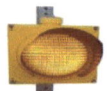

Moderate -score 6-10. This group can be managed by primary care professionals through counselling, such as brief intervention. They may or may not need help of an addiction specialist.

Mild- score 1-5. This group can be managed by primary care through brief intervention and motivational intervention counselling.

Concept Eight
Cobweb of Addiction

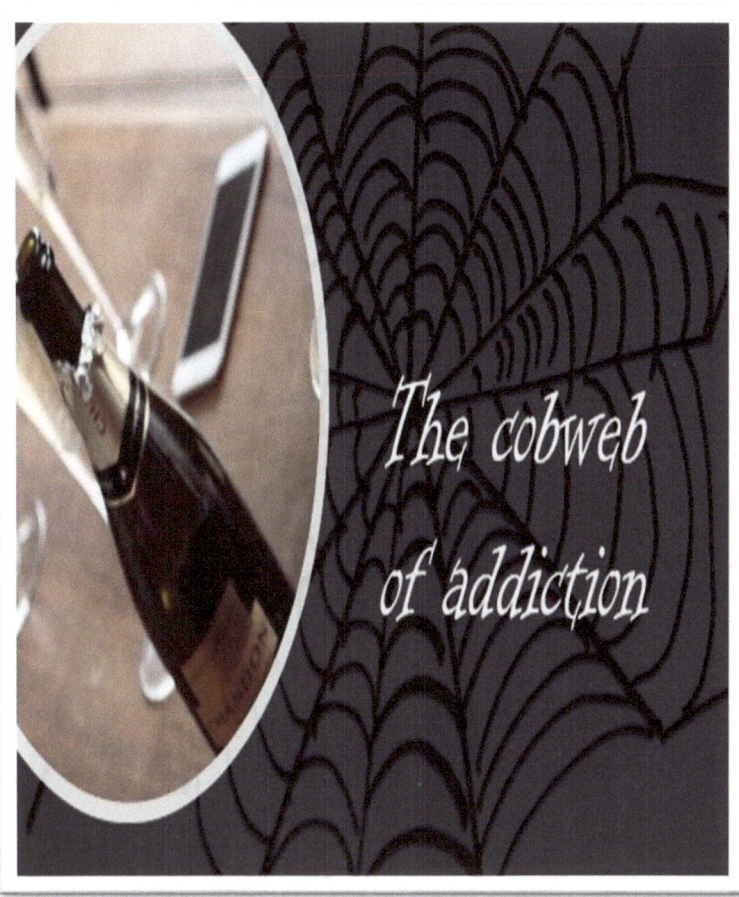

Unfortunately, the cobweb of addiction not only engulfs a person using a substance but also entangles the life of family members. The challenging aspect for substance users is to cope with the frustration of dependence. On the one hand, they want to cease the intake by their will power. On the other hand, the sign of withdrawal makes it impossible to stay away from the drug and alcohol. These easy to understand stories are written in a layman format to provide an overview of how person and family entrapped in the cobweb of addiction suffers almost daily.

www.ingramcontent.com/pod-product-compliance
Lightning Source LLC
Chambersburg PA
CBHW040316220526
45473CB00009B/2459